The Strain Strategist

Home Fitness for Weight Loss and Beyond":

Meta J. Myers

Copyright

Disclaimer

For basic informational reasons only, the data presented in "The Strain Strategist: Home Fitness for Weight Loss and Beyond" Any accidents, illnesses, or losses resulting from using the methods, exercises, or material in this book are not the responsibility of the author or publisher. Before beginning any new fitness program, it is best to speak with a healthcare provider, particularly if you have any underlying medical concerns. Any negative effects or repercussions arising from the use of the material in this book, whether direct or indirect, are disclaimed by the author and publisher.

Table of contents

INTRODUCTION

Hello and welcome to "The Strain Strategist: Home Fitness for Weight Loss and Beyond." This guide takes you on a trip to turn your house into a fitness haven while educating you about the dynamic world of resistance training and how important it is for both weight loss and general health.

You'll learn the fundamentals of efficient at-home exercises as we go through the following sections, from determining your current fitness level to choosing the appropriate resistance equipment. This article explains the importance of at-home exercise and offers tips for creating a customized training schedule that meets your objectives.

Get ready to enjoy intense exercises that train many muscle groups, improving not just your body but also your strength and stamina. To take your workout to the next level, we'll look at advanced tactics that combine weight training, cardio, and intensity training.

The trip doesn't stop with the physical; we'll explore the areas of stretching and recuperation, realizing the significance of flexibility and renewal in maintaining a long-term fitness quest. Nutritional advice will support your efforts and provide your body with the nutrition it needs to lose weight and succeed overall.

Any fitness journey will have challenges; we'll provide you with the tools to be persistent, get past obstacles, and acknowledge your accomplishments. You'll learn how home exercise promotes holistic well-being and lays a strong, long-lasting basis for a healthy lifestyle as we go beyond weight reduction.

This handbook serves as more than simply a reference; it's a traveling companion for success. Together, let's take this life-changing adventure to realize the full potential of at-home exercise and develop into your own Strain Strategist.

UNDERSTANDING THE IMPORTANCE OF HOME FITNESS

We will discuss the basic reasons that home exercise is an essential part of your overall health in this section. Here's a summary of the main ideas:

Practicality and Availability

•Talk about the ease of working out from home, removing obstacles such as commuting time and gym appointments.

•Put emphasis on how accessible at-home exercise is for people leading hectic lives.

Customized Setting

•Examine the advantages of designing a customized training area based on your tastes.

• Describe how motivation and consistency are fostered by a welcoming atmosphere.

Regularity and Extended-Term Dedication

•The significance of creating a regular exercise regimen in the comfortable environment of your home should be emphasized.

•Talk about how easily incorporating fitness into daily life makes long-term commitment more attainable.

The cost-effectiveness

• Examine the financial benefits that come with working out at home, such as the lack of gym memberships and travel costs.

•Consist in arguing that investing in the very minimum of equipment may produce satisfactory outcomes and make fitness affordable.

Comfort and Seclusion

• Discuss the privacy benefits of working out at home, targeting individuals who might feel uneasy in a public fitness facility.

•Talk about how having a comfortable environment of your own encourages a good outlook when working out.

Involvement of Family and Community

•Examine how family or community activities centered around home fitness might promote a common goal of well-being.

• Emphasize the possibility of establishing a home workout setting that is encouraging.

Gaining an appreciation for the importance of at-home exercise in your quest for a better lifestyle begins with comprehending these factors.

SETTING THE FOUNDATION

Let's take a moment to set the groundwork for your fitness journey before we go into intense workouts. This chapter serves as your architectural blueprint to make sure your home gym is a long-lasting structure. We'll talk about the following:

1. Comprehending "Strain": The Secret to Opening Doors

•Learn the science behind "strain" and why it's so important for promoting fat reduction, muscular growth, and overall fitness advancement.

• Acquire the skill of carefully applying strain to your workouts to maximize gains and reduce the chance of injury.

2.Attitude Matters: Learning to Overcome Obstacles, Maintain Motivation, and Form Long-Term Fitness Habits.

• Dive into the mental game of fitness and learn how to develop consistency and motivation.

•Find how to divert turning out from an errand into a cherished part of your life by figuring out how to make it fulfilling and pleasurable.

3.Setting Objectives: Choosing Your Path to Achievement

• Gain expertise in making Brilliant wellness targets, which represent exact, quantifiable, feasible, pertinent, and time-bound.

•To retain motivation and develop momentum, break big goals into smaller, more manageable tasks.

4.Putting Up Your Home Workout: Needed Equipment and Low-Cost Options

• Learn about the necessary gear for efficient at-home workouts, such as bodyweight training equipment, resistance bands, and optional extras.

•Inventive DIY substitutes and commonplace items may be used to outfit your home gym affordably.

5.Setting Up Your Area: Establishing a Comfortable Workout Setting

•Regardless of space limitations, discover how to use your home for effective and safe workouts.

•Discover strategies for reducing outside distractions and fostering an inspiring training environment.

6.Heating Up and Heating Down: Safeguarding Your Body and Improving Outcomes

• Learn how crucial good warm-ups and cool-downs are to preventing injuries, improving performance, and promoting recovery.

• Acquire knowledge of targeted warm-up and cool-down activities that complement different training styles.

By becoming proficient in these fundamentals, you'll position yourself for long-term success and guarantee the knowledge, drive, and careful preparation that forms the cornerstone of your at-home fitness journey. Remember that even the greatest athletic achievements begin with one step, and this is the first one.

ASSESSING YOUR FITNESS LEVEL

It's a good idea to snap a brief "fitness selfie" to gauge your current fitness level before throwing yourself into a workout. Merely a few straightforward observations and an honest evaluation of oneself will suffice:

1.Stair Power: What's the sensation of those steps? Do you use the elevator, huff and puff halfway up, or conquer them like a mountain goat? You can see a hint of your cardiovascular fitness by climbing stairs.

2.Bodyweight Buddies: How do the fundamental exercises of lunges, squats, and push-ups feel? Simple enough, a little difficult, or nearly impossible? These workouts highlight your general coordination and strength.

3.Daily Hustle: How busy are you when you're not working out? Do you spend most of your day sitting down, walking or biking small distances, or using the stairs? Your daily activity level affects how many calories you burn and how fit you are overall.

4.Rest & Recharge: How do you feel following simple tasks? Regaining your vitality or in need of a protracted nap? Progress depends on recovery, so observe how your body reacts to exertion.

5.Taking Notes on Your Body is Crucial! Any discomfort, aches, or limits? Show them some respect! To prevent injury, change up your workouts or take days off.

Recall that this is only the beginning. Remember that you are unique and shouldn't compare yourself to others. Make use of this knowledge to select exercises that are fun, safe, and productive for you.

Bonus tip: Monitor your advancement! Make notes or take photos so you can track your progress over time. Rewarding minor victories can help you stay inspired to continue your fitness journey!

CHOOSING THE RIGHT RESISTANCE EQUIPMENT

Consider resistance training gear as your go-to tool for toning muscle, increasing metabolism, and improving the quality of your at-home exercises. To help you select the appropriate equipment for your fitness objectives, consider the following brief guide:

1.Bands of resistance:

•Advantages: Adaptable to varying strength levels, lightweight, portable, and reasonably priced.

•Excellent for: Mobility work, rehab, strength training, toning, and full-body workouts.

•Advice: To advance as you gain strength, use bands with different resistance levels (light, medium, and heavy).

2.Body Mass:

The benefits include testing your core and coordination, not requiring any special equipment, and being portable.

•Excellent for: Enhancing balance, increasing functional strength, and burning calories.
•Advice: To provide variation and intensity, utilize everyday objects like chairs, stairs, or water bottles.

3.Kettlebells and dumbbells are free weights.

•Benefits: Classic for enhancing muscle and strength; targets particular muscle regions.

•Excellent for: Muscle isolation, strength training, and compound workouts.

•Advice: Practice with lesser weights until you have perfected your form, then go on to heavier ones.

4.Tubes with resistance:

•Advantages: Handles add additional grip possibilities; otherwise, similar to bands.

•Excellent for upper body workouts, rehabilitation, strength training, and toning.

•For further exercise diversity, use door anchors.

Athletic Suspension:

•Advantages: Adaptable, demanding, and activating several muscle groups simultaneously.

•Excellent for: Functional training, full-body exercises, and strengthening the core.

•A solid anchor point is essential for a secure installation.

Keep in mind:

•Commence with something basic: To start, select one or two types of equipment.

•Think of your objectives: Make sure the equipment you select meets your fitness goals.

•Honor your personal space: Select exercise equipment that works for your space.

•Pay attention to your body and select equipment that is both joint-safe and pleasant.

Enjoy your time experimenting! Enjoy the process and figure out what works best for you!

WEIGHT LOSS ESSENTIALS

So you need to get in shape and shed a couple of pounds? Fantastic! However, remember that eating regimens or quick fixes aren't the way to long-haul weight reduction. It is about developing long-lasting, health-conscious habits. This is your go-to guide for the fundamentals:

1.Eat sensibly, for the most part.

•Don't feed your cravings—fuel your body! Consider whole grains, fruits, vegetables, lean meat, and healthy fats. Give up processed meals, sugar-filled beverages, and large servings.

•Don't starve yourself; give yourself the odd treat. Moderation is essential since deprivation breeds binges!

•Stay hydrated like a pro—water is on your side. Try to have eight glasses a day to stay satiated and avoid feeling full.

2.Move your body and enjoy yourself!

•Locate things you like doing: It doesn't matter if you're walking, dancing, swimming, or biking—just get moving!

•Start small and expand over time; consistency is essential. Spend 20 minutes a day, three to four times a week, and progressively increase the time and intensity.

•Accept at-home exercise: Not a gym? Not a problem! You can work out like a pro with bodyweight exercises, resistance bands, and internet videos.

Rest well and reduce stress:

•Make sleep a priority: Attempt to get 7–8 hours every night. Hormones that influence weight are disturbed by sleep deprivation.

•Reduce stress by finding relaxing activities like yoga, meditation, or time spent in nature. Stress may be the catalyst for adverse eating habits.

3.Treat yourself with kindness.

•Enjoy the little victories. Losing a pound or starting a new exercise regimen is a success!

•Prioritize progress over perfection. There will be hiccups on the road. Don't allow obstacles to stop you. Just get back on course!

•Pay attention to your body. Take breaks when necessary, and challenge yourself when prepared. It's your trip; change course if necessary.

Recall that losing weight is a marathon, not a sprint. You'll be well on your way to being a better, happier version of yourself if you make these fundamentals a regular habit!

Bonus advice: enlist help! For individualized advice, find a workout partner, sign up for an online community, or consult a qualified dietician.

THE ROLE OF RESISTANCE TRAINING IN WEIGHT LOSS

Forget self-starvation or never-ending cardio! Resistance exercise is a weight reduction secret weapon that is readily apparent. Here's the lowdown on why gaining muscle is the best way to lose weight:

1.The Metabolic Marvel, Muscle:

•Consider your muscles as your furnace for burning calories. The more you have, the more fuel your body burns, even when at rest! This means that you are always burning fat!

•Building and strengthening muscle using weights, bands, or your own body weight with resistance training increases metabolism and helps you burn calories long after your workout.

2.Beyond Measuring

•Losing weight is about more than simply the weight on the scale. Resistance training gives you a toned, muscular figure by helping to mold your body.

•Although you won't lose weight as rapidly as you would on a restrictive diet, you will grow muscle, burn fat, and feel stronger and more confident about your appearance.

3.Extra Advantages:

•Better balance, better posture, and stronger bones are just a few benefits of weight exercise.

•It also elevates your energy and attitude, giving you a positive, whole-body feeling!

4.Begin Small, Grow Larger:

•A gym membership or expensive equipment are not necessary. You may begin with bodyweight workouts, resistance bands, or even soup cans.

•As you gain strength, gradually increase the duration and intensity of your workouts from manageable starting points.

Recall:

To see results, persistence and time are required. Remain focused, have patience, and relish the process!

For the best results in terms of weight loss and general fitness, combine resistance training with a nutritious diet and frequent exercise.

CREATING AN EFFECTIVE HOME WORKOUT PLAN

converting your living room to a gym? This is your how-to manual for creating a fun, efficient, and consistently rewarding at-home exercise program!

1.Determine Your Objective:

•Fat Blaster: Use interval training, which combines brief rest intervals with burst activities, to burn calories and speed your metabolism. Consider burpees, lunges, and jumping jacks!

•Muscle Sculptor: Resistance exercise helps to tone and build muscle in the body. Reach for some training bands and dumbbells, or utilize ordinary household objects like water bottles in a novel way!

•Cardio Cruiser: Engaging in physical activities such as swimming, dancing, or jogging can increase heart rate and improve endurance. Simply move your body; no specialized equipment is required!

2.Mix and Match Frenzy:

• Maintain variety: Avoid becoming stale! To keep your body engaged and your workouts interesting, switch up your repertoire of bodyweight exercises, strength training, and cardiovascular activities.

• Pay attention to your body: Plan days of relaxation and avoid exerting yourself while you're hurt. Recall: it's about progress, not perfection!

•Short and Sweet: Lacking hours? Make time for three to four 20–30 minute workouts per week. The secret is to be consistent!

3.Take it as Yours:

• Select enjoyable activities: dance your way to health with Zumba or get together with a friend for an online exercise dance party! Having fun inspires motivation.

• Use your imagination: Not able to perform push-ups? Adapt while on your knees! Not even a treadmill? Scale those steps! Look for strategies to adapt exercise to your needs.

•Music Matters: Play energetic songs that make you want to move and get your heart rate up!

4.Extra Advice:

•Warm up and cool down: Before and after each workout, stretch your body gently to prepare it and avoid injuries.

• Monitor your advancement: Honor your victories! Recognizing your accomplishments, whether it's learning a new workout or surpassing your personal best, keeps you inspired.

• Join the group: Apps for exercising and online fitness clubs provide motivation, encouragement, and virtual training partners!

Keep in mind that your at-home exercise regimen is your own private playground. Make it enjoyable, productive, and most of all, something you truly love! Put on your sneakers, turn up the music, and get ready to dominate your living room gym because you are the boss of your fitness journey!

DYNAMIC WORKOUTS

Put an end to monotonous exercises and repetitions! The exciting and effective dynamic exercises are here to add to your fitness journey. Imagine your body becoming a symphony of motion, moving fluidly and in a continual flow. In a word, that is dynamic training.

How Do Dynamic Workouts Work?

These exercises replace regulated motions and static holds with continuous, deliberate movements. Consider high knees, twisting lunges, jumping jacks, and other exercises that require your body to move in many planes of motion.

For what Reason Are They Dynamic?

•Metabolic Pandemonium: You might build your digestion and consume more calories even after you've quit sweating by keeping a raised pulse and contracted muscles during your exercise.

•Portability Expert: Counting dynamic stretches into your activity will expand your scope of movement, adaptability, and readiness, which will assist you with moving more smoothly and with more prominent coordination.

•Injury Inhibitor: By moving your joints and muscles to warm them up and prepare your body for the demands of exercise, you can lower your risk of injury.

Fun Factor: Let's be honest, performing static workouts may get boring. Fitness becomes more of a game and less of a duty when you do dynamic exercises since they are entertaining, captivating, and keep you on your toes (literally!).

Workouts that are Dynamic Examples:

•Interval Circuits: Switch between medium-intensity recovery exercises, like jumping jacks, and high-intensity workouts, like burpees.

•Animal Flow: For a novel and difficult exercise, try moving like bears, monkeys, or crabs.

•Yoga Flow: Arrange flowing yoga poses in a rhythmic, heart-pounding sequence.

•Plyometrics: To develop explosive power and speed, explode into lunges, squats, and leaps.

Customizing it to Yourself:

•Begin with basics: Start with simple exercises and work your way up to more difficult and intense ones.

•Be Innovative: Create your own dynamic sequences with resistance bands, household items, and your bodyweight.

•Pay Attention to Your Body: Adjust workouts as necessary, and take days off when necessary.

•To find your flow, follow the beat of your own movement and savor the sensation of your body moving.

Exercises that are dynamic can lead to a fitness journey that is more enjoyable, productive, and injury-free. Enter the flow, let loose your inner movers, and experience the invigorating force of dynamic fitness!

FULL-BODY STRAIN SESSIONS

Ignore isolated exercises that focus on certain muscular groups. Explore the world of full-body strain sessions, where each exercise is a masterful fusion of coordinated motion that will test your limitations and ignite your most profound sources of strength and endurance.

Full-Body Strain Sessions: What Are They?

These workouts aren't your normal ones. They are painstakingly constructed circuits intended to:

•In every exercise, use every muscle group, from your fingers to your toes.

• Put your cardiovascular system through its paces to keep your heart rate up and your body burning calories like a fire.

•Demand courage, drive, and mental toughness to push beyond exhaustion.

Develop practical strength by simulating everyday motions to create a physique that is prepared for anything.

Why Stress?: The Covert Tool

"Strain" does not mean forcing oneself to fail. It all comes down to identifying that sweet spot when your muscles are just ready to give up and push themselves to get stronger. This specific stress increases metabolism, stimulates muscular growth, and shapes a toned, slender body.

Full-body strain session examples include:

• Tabata Torture: Perform burpees, sprints, or mountain climbers for 20 seconds at maximum effort, followed by 10 seconds of recovery, eight times. Get ready to perspire!

•AMRAP Mayhem: Perform as many AMRAP repetitions (AMRAP) of the following five exercises in five minutes: squats, lunges, push-ups, rows, and jumps. Repeat three times while feeling the burn get stronger.

•Partner Playtime: For activities like medicine ball tosses, push-ups with hand claps, and partner squats, pair up with a friend. The healthy rivalry challenges you both to greater heights.

• Bodyweight Buffet: Perform exercises like bench dips, inverted rows from a bar, and lunges with jumping jacks using just your body weight. Easy to use, yet remarkably powerful.

Opening Up the Whole-Body Strain:

•Start Small: Select workouts that you can do with proper technique. Intensify and increase complexity as you gain strength.

• Vary Your Circuits: Change up your workouts, rep ranges, and recovery times to keep your body guessing.

• Pay Attention to Your Body: Adjust workouts to avoid injury and take breaks as necessary.

•Accept the Burn: Keep in mind that while a strain is momentary, the effects are long-lasting. Embrace the progress and persevere through the discomfort.

Sessions involving full body strain are not recommended for the timid. They are for those who are eager to sculpt a physique that is both powerful and attractive, who are hungry for a challenge, and who want to release their inner beast. Enter the ring aware of your limitations, and be ready to win your fitness contest.

TARGETED MUSCLE GROUPS: ARMS, LEGS, CORE

Are you prepared to define some areas and achieve more power and definition? Greetings from the world of focused muscular training! Arms, legs, and core are the movement powerhouses that will be our main emphasis. Now let's get into the specifics of creating each zone:

Arms:

• Curls of all kinds—barbell, dumbbell, hammer, and concentration—build those gunslingers and blast those biceps. Remember to perform pull-ups and chin-ups to fully activate your biceps.

•Tricep Toners: To give your arms a chiseled appearance, tone and shape your triceps with push-ups of all kinds, dips, overhead presses, and tricep extensions.

•Forearm Fury: Pay attention to these unsung champions of strength! Rock-solid forearms are developed through grip challenges, farmer's carries, and wrist curls, which enhance performance in all workouts.

Legs:

•Quad Commanders: Squats are the ultimate leg-builders, available in a variety of magnificent forms like bodyweight, weighted, jump, and split squats. Lunges and leg presses provide variation and focus on certain quadriceps.

•Hamstring Heroes: For sculpted hamstrings, which are necessary for forceful movement and injury prevention, try deadlifts, Romanian deadlifts, hamstring curls, and glute bridges.

•Calf Crusher: Any type of calf raise, whether performed on a step, while seated or standing, will give your calves the definition they deserve and enhance your agility and balance.

Central Champions:

•Plank Perfection: By using your complete core with high, low, side, and leg lift variants, you may improve strength and stability from your diaphragm to your lower back.

•Crunch Crew: Make sure you perform crunches! Certain core muscles are targeted by traditional, bicycle, reverse, and Russian twists, which help to shape and strengthen your midsection.

•Anti-Rotation Activators: By testing your core's capacity to withstand twisting forces, exercises like side planks, dead bugs, and anti-rotation presses help to improve your posture and general stability.

Recall:

•Warm-up and cool-down: Always warm up and cool down with appropriate workouts to prepare your muscles and avoid injury.

•Progressive overload: To maintain pushing your muscles and promoting growth, gradually increase the weight, repetitions, or sets.

• Form is everything: Put good form before bigger weights. A well-executed bodyweight squat is preferable than a careless one performed with large weights.

• Pay attention to your body: Adjust workouts and take breaks as necessary to prevent damage.

• Maintaining balance: Don't ignore your other muscle groups. For a well-rounded fitness regimen, incorporate aerobic and full-body exercises into your regimen.

You may build the body of your dreams by carefully focusing on your arms, legs, and core. So pick up some weights, go on your mat, and tackle every obstacle on your path to health! Recall that throughout this journey, perseverance, commitment, and appropriate form are your allies. Prepare to let loose your inner carpenter and create a physique that is powerful, toned, and prepared for anything.

ADVANCED STRATEGIES

Congratulations! You've overcome plateaus, learned the fundamentals, and now your regular exercises seem almost like a habit. Do not be alarmed, fighter of fitness! It's time to use these cutting-edge techniques to get to the next level:

1.Power of Periodization:

•Spread It Out: Get Rid of the Same O.S. To keep your body guessing and maximize results, alternate between high intensity, strength development, and endurance training phases throughout your exercises.

•Supercharge Sets: Push yourself with drop sets, which include decreasing weight while increasing repetitions within a set, or supersets, which combine two exercises back-to-back.

•Volume Variations: Depending on your current objective, experiment with sets, repetitions, and rest intervals to discover the sweet spot for strength, endurance, or muscular growth.

2.Overcoming Muscle Mind:

• Illustration Triumph: See it to realize it! Imagine yourself finishing that lengthy run or mastering that difficult activity. Performance and confidence are enhanced by mental rehearsal.

•Mind-Muscle Connection: During each exercise, pay attention to the particular muscle you're exercising. This maximizes focused growth and strengthens the bond.

•Meditation for Motivation: Increase your pre-exercise focus and fight workout jitters by practicing mindfulness techniques like meditation.

3.Adding Fuel to the Fire:

•Tweaks to Carb Timing: Try timing your carbohydrate intake to coincide with your exercise. carbohydrates before an exercise might provide you energy, and carbohydrates after a workout can help you recuperate.

•Hydration Hero: Staying properly hydrated isn't limited to hot weather. Try to drink the same amount of water every day to maintain muscular function and peak performance.

•Slumber for Strength: Never undervalue the power of a good night's sleep! Make getting 7-8 hours of good sleep a priority for your body's healing of muscles, replenishment of energy, and hormonal balance.

3.Accept the Community:

• Discover Your Tribe: Join like-minded fitness enthusiasts for training! For inspiration and encouragement, locate a workout partner, enroll in a group class, or communicate online.

• Track Your success: To keep track of your success, utilize fitness apps or keep a training record. Observing the fruits of your labor increases motivation and aids in the improvement of your tactics.

•Seek Expert Guidance: For individualized training regimens, technique correction, and advice on cutting-edge approaches, think about collaborating with a certified trainer or coach.

Recall that sophisticated tactics are precisely that: sophisticated. Don't dive in headfirst without a good foundation and the right advice. Take care of your body, look for assistance, and most of all, enjoy yourself! Peak fitness is a journey, not a destination, that requires constant investigation. Savor the journey, accept the difficulties, and marvel at the amazing things your body is capable of.

INTENSITY TECHNIQUES FOR ACCELERATED RESULTS

Consider your exercise routine as a bonfire. It's necessary to fan the flames sometimes in order to make them roar. This is where intensity training methods come in handy; they act as fuel for your fitness fire, assisting you with:

• Increase caloric expenditure

• Gain muscle more quickly

• Get above obstacles

• Put yourself through emotional and physical strain

The following are a few of the best intensity techniques:

1. Supersets

•Exercises like squats and pull-ups may be combined back-to-back to target various muscle areas.

•Maintain an elevated heart rate and continuous muscular contraction.

2. Sets of Drops:

•After completing a set to failure, immediately lower the weight and perform further repetitions.

•Work your muscles as hard as possible.

3. Take a Break:

•During a set, take quick rest intervals of 10 to 20 seconds to enable you to lift bigger weights for more repetitions.

•boosts the power and strength of muscles.

4. Drawbacks:

•Concentrate on the exercise's lowering phase, reducing the weight gradually and under control for three to five seconds.

•increases muscular endurance and strength.

5. HIIT, or High-Intensity Interval Training:

•Switch between quick bursts of maximal exertion and few rest intervals.

•increases cardiovascular fitness and burns calories.

6. Tabata:

•a particular type of high-intensity interval training (HIIT) that consists of four minutes of 20 seconds of intensive work and 10 seconds of relaxation.

•A simple and efficient technique to increase metabolism and push your boundaries.

Recall:

Intensive approaches are not appropriate for novices. Prior to adding them, have a strong base in fitness.

• Recognize your body's needs and take pauses when necessary. A result of overtraining is injury.

• Use intensity training methods sparingly—not during every workout.

•For best effects, combine them with appropriate diet and recuperation.

Use intensity strategies to kickstart your fitness journey, but don't forget to put safety, form, and listening to your body's signals first at all times. Take on the task, feel the intensity, and watch as your fitness level soars!

INCORPORATING CARDIO WITH RESISTANCE

Do you believe that in the realm of fitness, weight training and cardio should be archrivals? Rethink that! It's like putting Captain Strength and Commander Cardio together to take on your fitness objectives when these two titans work together. This is the reason why:

1.Increasing Fat Burning:

•Building Muscle: Resistance exercise increases muscle mass, and increased muscle mass increases calorie expenditure even during rest. Cardio becomes even more efficient at burning fat as a result.

•Double Burn Bonanza: You may burn calories for hours by including cardio intervals into your resistance training or by performing a cardio session after lifting weights.

2.Creating an Equilibrium Body:

•Strength Meets Stamina: Resistance training increases muscular tone and strength while cardiovascular exercise improves heart health and endurance. Together, you'll become a champion of well-rounded fitness who can handle everything.

•Partners in Injury Prevention: Robust muscles enhance body awareness and support your joints, lowering your chance of injury when engaging in aerobic activities.

3.Keeping Things Novel:

•Avoid the Boredom Binge by alternating between weightlifting and swimming, dancing, or jogging.

•You won't go into a fitness slump since your body and mind will remain active.

•Test Every System: By varying your exercises, you may prevent plateaus and experience faster results since your body will continue to adapt and grow.

How to Merge Like a Pro:

•Start Easy: Before introducing weights or vigorous exercise, if you're new to it, start with bodyweight exercises and gentle cardio.

• Pay Attention to Your Body: Don't overdo it and take breaks when needed. Recall that maintaining consistency is more important than working oneself to the bone.

•Find Your Balance: Try out various aerobic and weight training combinations and durations to see what suits you and your objectives the best.

Bonus Advice: Have fun! Pick something you like doing, like dancing alone in your living room, going on a hike with friends, or taking a group fitness class.

So let go of the competition over fitness and enjoy the strength of the combination. To maximize its potential, your body needs the dynamic combination of resistance and cardio exercise. Prepare to experience an unprecedented level of strength, fitness, and vigor!

RECOVERY AND STRETCHING

It feels perfect to stretch yourself to the edge at the rec center, yet in the event that you don't extend and recuperate appropriately, you're getting yourself in a position for disappointment. Envision that extending and restoration are the daylight and water that an exerciser needs to bloom into serious areas of strength for a plant. Exercise is like sowing that seed.

Recuperation: Fill up and Recreate

• **Sleep is King (or Queen):** To allow your muscles to heal and your mind to refresh, try to get 7-8 hours of good sleep each night. Sleep deprivation is akin to equipping a Ferrari with a rusted engine.

•**Fuel Up Wisely**: To refill nutrients and energy storage, fuel your body with wholesome meals and lots of water. Consider consuming carbohydrates to restore energy and protein to heal muscles.

• **Active Healing:** It is possible to reduce physical strain and improve circulation by recovering through gentle activities like swimming, yoga, or walking. Going for a comfortable stroll is desirable over relaxing on the love seat

• **Pay Attention to Your Body**: Pain is not natural, but soreness is. When necessary, take rest days and avoid pushing yourself past discomfort.Focus on your body's signs and give it the rest it expects to appropriately work. Stretching: Increasing Length and Power

• **Dynamic Warm-Up:** Use mild exercises like jumping jacks, arm circles, and leg swings to prepare your muscles and get your blood flowing before your workout. Think of it as gently waking up your body after getting out of bed.

• **Static Stretches:** To expand the scope of movement and adaptability, hold for 30 to 60 seconds following an exercise. Really focus on your back, quads, and hamstrings. Imagine it as a profound tissue knead for your muscles.

• **Versatility Sorcery**: Incorporate versatility-upgrading developments like spine turns, hip circles, and shoulder rolls to expand the scope of movement in your joints. Envision it as the way into your body's idle potential.

Try not to skip it. Despite the fact that extending may not be the most exciting activity, it's fundamental for lessening the risk of injury, improving execution, and having a decent outlook on your body. Take it in the same vein as brushing your teeth: assuming that you do it every day, you'll obtain improved results!

Recovering and stretching are crucial components of your fitness journey; they are not optional extras. You'll make sure your body is prepared to function at its peak, prevent injuries, and feel fantastic all along the road by giving them priority. Accept the positive and negative aspects of fitness, and you'll see rapid development!

Bonus Advice: Look for methods to add enjoyment to stretching and recuperation. Stretch while listening to soothing music, take a soothing bath with Epsom salts, or work on it with a buddy to get some company. Make it a ritual you eagerly anticipate rather than a task to do!

IMPORTANCE OF RECOVERY IN HOME FITNESS

Consider your at-home exercises as sowing the seeds of your strength and health. However, for these seeds to really thrive, the same conditions must be met as in any garden. What is the element that's kept a secret? recuperation. It goes beyond simply relaxing on the sofa, though that is always good (some well-earned downtime!). To fully benefit from your sweat sessions, recovery requires the sunshine and water that feed your body and mind.

The Significance of Rehabilitation

• **Muscle Magic**: Your muscles are repairing themselves after a workout. They get the energy and time they need to rebuild stronger and leaner with rest and a healthy diet. If you put off recovering, you run the danger of becoming hurt or falling behind.

• **Energy Oasis:** Excessive exertion depletes your energy stores. Refueling your body with nutritious foods, relaxation days, and adequate sleep can leave you feeling reenergized and prepared to take on your next workout.

•**Mind Matters**: Engaging in exercise may also be psychologically taxing. Your mind may relax, concentrate, and become more motivated and focused when you return to your exercises after a period of recovery.

Hacks for Recuperation for Home Fitness Pioneers:

•**Sleep Sanctuary:** Try to get seven to eight hours of good sleep every night. It's like putting your body and mind on vacation.

• **Eat Wisely**: To recharge your muscles and offer energy for recuperation, choose wholesome meals full of protein, carbohydrates, and healthy fats. Consider a smoothie after working out, whole-wheat bread with avocado, or a vegetable omelet.

• **Hydration Hero**: Make water your ally! To keep your body working at its best and to flush out toxins, stay hydrated during the day and after exercise.

•**Stretching Symphony**: Light stretches make you feel good about your body, avoid muscular tension, and increase flexibility after a workout and on rest days. Consider it a calming orchestra for your musculature.

•**Relaxation & Rest**: Never undervalue the importance of relaxation! When you need a day off, take it and engage in your favorite hobbies, such as reading, taking a bath, or spending time with close friends and family. Allow your body and mind to experience true relaxation.

Recuperation is about being strategic, not just being slothful. It will make you stronger, healthier, and happier if you make it a priority. So enjoy the downtime, replenish your energy, and watch as your at-home exercise endeavor soars!

Bonus Advice: Look for methods to appreciate your recuperation. Make a soothing post-workout routine, stretch to soothing music, or go for a stroll in the outdoors. Make it a ritual you eagerly anticipate rather than a task to do!

STRETCHING FOR FLEXIBILITY AND INJURY PREVENTION

Imagine your body as a well-maintained machine. It requires every component to operate smoothly and to the fullest extent possible in order for it to function at its peak. This is where stretching comes in handy; it's like having WD-40 for your muscles—it keeps them flexible, loose, and prepared for anything.

Why 8 You Stretch to Reach Fitness Success?

• **Flexibility Fiesta**: A greater range of motion is possible for your joints and muscles when you have good flexibility. This enhances your posture, facilitates daily tasks, and gives you greater strength and grace in your movements.

• **Injury Interceptor**: Consider taut muscles as potential injury time bombs. Frequent stretching releases this tension, lowers your chance of sprains, pulls, and pains, and keeps you competitive.

•**Performance Pump**: Your muscles function more effectively when they aren't entirely tense. Better form, better outcomes, and even breaking past those annoying plateaus are all a result of this.

Stretching Made Easy:

• **Get warmed up Sensibly**: Avoid stretching chilled muscles! Warm up your muscles and blood moving with some mild aerobics or dynamic stretches like arm circles or leg swings.

•**Static Serenity:** Hold mild stretches for 30 to 60 seconds after working out or on days when you're taking a break.

•Pay special attention to your back, quads, and hamstrings. Keep in mind that here, smooth and slow wins the race!

• **Pay Attention to Your Body**: Gain without suffering! Stop immediately if a stretch feels painful or sharp. Respect your body's limitations and ease yourself into it.

•**Buddy Up**: It may be inspiring and enjoyable to stretch with a friend! One person can maintain a position while the other checks forms. Sharing the laughter and perspiration also helps it to feel less like a chore.

Bonus advice: Make it a daily routine to stretch. You can even do it while waiting for your coffee to brew, watching TV, or listening to music. Yoga gets more useful and natural the more you incorporate it into your routine.

And remember, stretching is more than just touching your toes (though that's good too!). It's about nourishing your body, realizing its maximum potential, and avoiding accidents. Thus, embrace the stretch, maintain your looseness, and use enjoyment and flexibility to achieve your exercise objectives!

NUTRITION TIPS FOR SUCCESS

Put an end to rigid regulations and convoluted diets! It's possible to nourish your body in a tasty, easy, and incredibly efficient way for fitness achievement. Here are a few simple strategies to keep your engine running:

•**Think Food, Not Fuel:** Adopt the mindset of "train to eat," rather than "eat to train." Food is more than simply exercise fuel—it's your body's companion. Savor a variety of delectable meals and snacks that fulfill your cravings and advance your objectives.

• **Maintaining Balance**: Aim for a colorful dish! Consume a lot of fruits and vegetables for fiber, vitamins, and minerals; whole grains for long-term energy; and lean protein for the repair of muscles. You also have buddies in nuts and avocados, which are healthy fats!

• **Hydration Hero**: Your greatest ally is water! Eight glasses should be consumed each day, or more if you perspire a lot. To stay constantly hydrated, give up sugar-filled beverages and carry a reusable water bottle with you at all times.

• **Snack Wisely**: Refrain from letting hunger stop you. Arrange nutritious munchies such as trail mix, vegetable sticks with hummus, or yogurt with berries. Steer clear of processed junk food and restrict your portion amounts.

• **Mindful Eating**: Indulge in your food! Eat mindfully of your hunger cues, chew everything completely, and take your time. Put an end to when you're full, not stuffed. Controlling portions and improving general health are aided by mindful eating.

• **Cook More, Stress Less:** Take some time to prepare meals instead of ordering takeout. Cooking is a joyful and fulfilling activity that gives you control over ingredients and amounts. Making a nutritious dinner is also a fantastic way to unwind.

• Delightful Candies In a strategic sense, avoid demonizing sweets! Eat them sometimes as snacks, but in moderation. For a well-balanced treat, go for smaller servings, handmade varieties, and mix them with fruit or yogurt.

• **Pay Attention to Your Body**: Everybody has unique demands. Observe how your body responds to different meals and modify your diet appropriately. Try a few different things and see what suits you the best.

•**There is no one-size-fits-all formula for nutrition**. These are only suggestions; feel free to adapt them to suit your requirements, interests, and objectives. Recall that eating well shouldn't be stressful; it should be pleasurable. Make wise decisions, feed your body with delectable foods, and watch as your fitness adventure takes off!

Bonus Advice: Have fun! Try out new dishes, investigate other culinary traditions, and include your loved ones in your quest for a balanced diet. You are more inclined to persevere through the procedure if you find it enjoyable.

FUELING YOUR BODY FOR WEIGHT LOSS

Put an end to headaches from calorie counting and crash diets! Giving your body the correct nourishment and paying attention to its needs will help you lose weight. Consider food as your ally, not your enemy, helping you to become a lighter, healthier version of yourself. Here's how to go about it:

1. Let Go of the Deprivation: Strict diets never work, leaving you disappointed and more ravenous than before. Rather, concentrate on plenty by consuming an abundance of nutritious grains, fruits, and veggies to keep you feeling content and full. Imagine vibrant salads, soups loaded with vegetables, and avocado on whole-wheat bread.

2. Protein Power: Even while you're at rest, your metabolism is boosted by lean protein, which aids in muscle growth and repair. To feel full and resist cravings, choose foods like Greek yogurt, grilled chicken, fish, beans, and lentils.

3. Fiber Frenzy: If you want to lose weight, fiber is your greatest buddy. By extending your sense of fullness, it helps you avoid mid-afternoon snacking episodes. For a fiber fiesta, pile your plate high with whole grains, broccoli, Brussels sprouts, and berries.

4. Hydration Hero: Your hidden weapon is water! Dehydration can cause your body to confuse thirst with appetite. Reusable water bottles are great for staying hydrated and reducing excessive eating. Keep one by your side and sip throughout the day.

5. Portion Perfection: The amount you consume matters just as much as what you eat. Measure portions, use smaller plates, and pay attention to your body's fullness signals. Put an end to when you're full, not stuffed.

6. Mindful Eating: Indulge in your food! Chew slowly and completely, savoring the flavors and sensations. Eating mindfully enables you to enjoy your meal, refrain from overindulging, and choose healthier options.

7. Sleep for Strength: Your body desires unhealthy meals and retains extra fat when you don't get enough sleep. To keep your hormones in check and your weight reduction progressing as planned, aim for 7-8 hours of good sleep per night.

8. Move Your Body: Exercise is essential for losing weight, but it doesn't have to involve strenuous long-distance running and boot camps. Make regular time for enjoyable activities such as dance, swimming, or brisk walks in your daily routine.

9. Give Up on Diet Mentality: Losing weight isn't about following rigid guidelines or fast remedies. It concerns a shift to a sustainable way of living. Prioritize eating a balanced diet, developing healthy habits, and acknowledging little accomplishments.

10. Pay Attention to Your Body: Everybody has unique demands. Observe the signals that your body is giving you.Make necessary changes to your diet and workout regimen if you feel lethargic or depleted.

Recall that feeding your body to lose weight does not entail starvation or punishment. It's about feeling well, making wise decisions, and relishing the ride. Accept a balanced, healthful lifestyle, pay attention to your body, and watch the weight drop off in a sustainable and organic way.

Bonus Advice: Have fun! Together with your friends, prepare vibrant meals, experiment with new, healthful dishes, and treat yourself to non-scale successes like more energy or better sleep. You're more likely to persevere and accomplish your objectives if you find the process enjoyable!

ROLE OF NUTRITION IN YOUR FITNESS JOURNEY

Consider your quest for fitness as a drive by car to the summit of a mountain. Your vehicle? Your form. Nutrition is the fuel!

Why does it matter so much?

•**Power Plant**: Food provides your body with the energy it needs to accomplish any task, including overcoming challenging workouts and recovering from exhausting sessions. Consider protein as your engine oil, carbohydrates as your gas, and healthy fats as your lubrication for the roads.

•**Building Blocks**: Protein functions as bricks, mending and constructing muscle to give you the strength and self-assurance to climb those hills.

•**Injury Interceptor**: Eating a healthy diet preserves your body in peak condition, which lowers the possibility of malfunctions and diversions that might keep you from working out.

• **Mental Magic:** Consuming a healthy diet also feeds your brain, which helps you stay motivated and focused when things become hard.

How can you now refuel for success?

Why Diversity Is Essential: Consider a rainbow platter! Include a variety of vibrant fruits and vegetables in your meals to provide vitamins, minerals, and energy to keep going.

•**Protein Power**: Don't cut corners on this fuel for growing muscle! Your allies on the path to a healthier you are lean meats, seafood, legumes, and nuts.

• **Hydration Hero**: Your hidden weapon is water! Drink enough water both before and throughout your ascent to keep your body and mind in top condition.

• **Mindful Eating**: Don't merely fill up automatically. To make smart decisions that keep you energized, savor your meal, pay attention to your body's hunger cues, and refrain from emotional eating.

• **Arrange for Smooth Travels**: Prevent hangover tantrums by carrying wholesome food for unforeseen diversions. Consider hummus on vegetable sticks, nuts, or fruits.

Recall that there is no one-size-fits-all dietary plan. Try new things, pay attention to your body, and discover what best feeds your own engine. Savor the trip, acknowledge your accomplishments, and observe as your fitness mountain descends beneath your resolute steps!

Bonus Advice: Have fun! Cook with friends, experiment with new recipes, and make eating well an experience. Reaching your peak becomes simpler the more fun you have in the process!

OVERCOMING CHALLENGES

Everybody has difficulties; those annoying impediments to achieving their objectives. But do not be alarmed, fellow explorer! Here's your basic toolbox to help you defeat them:

Modify Your Perspective:

•Problem: "This isn't feasible!"

•Shift: "This is tough, but I can learn and grow."

By shifting your viewpoint from one of failure to one of opportunity, you may approach problems with a solution-focused mindset.

Dissect it:

•Difficulty: "It's too big!"

•Move: "I can walk a little distance."

Are you feeling overpowered? Divide the challenge into more manageable tasks. One manageable objective at a time!

Seek Assistance:

•Ask yourself: "I'm alone."
•Shift: "I can get assistance."

Alone, no one climbs mountains. Speak with loved ones, mentors, coworkers, or experts.

Their support and direction might serve as your climbing rope.

Accept Errors:

•Admit defeat: "I failed."

•Shift: "I learned and I'll try again."

Errors are not fatalities; rather, they are stepping stones. Examine what went wrong, modify your strategy, and proceed still.

Honor Your Wins:

•Prompt: "I'm stuck."

•Say to yourself, "I've come this far!"

Recognize your accomplishments, no matter how tiny. Enjoying small or large victories helps you stay focused and motivated.

Pay Attention to the Here and Now:

•Daunting assertion: "The future is scary."

•Shift: "I am now responsible for my actions.

You won't be able to climb the mountain by worrying about the future. Pay attention to the current work and the steps you are taking.

Recall:

•You underestimate your strength.

•Difficulties provide chances for growth and learning.

•Every little bit of progress counts as a win.

So, traveler, arm yourself with this basic equipment, take on your obstacles head-on, and summit that peak!

Bonus Tip: Embrace the comedy in the ascent! Even on the toughest days, you may stay upbeat and cheerful by laughing at your mistakes and yourself.

CONSISTENT WITH HOME WORKOUTS

Workouts at home are fantastic! What's not to love? No crowds, flexible scheduling, and the ability to dance in your jammies. To be honest, though, maintaining consistency may sometimes seem like squaring up a very slick octopus. Fear not, fighter of fitness! Here are a few easy ideas to make your living room a regular (and enjoyable!) workout area:

1.Locate Your Fire:

•Passion Power: Choose pursuits that you sincerely love! Doing bodyweight circuits, yoga, or dancing help you move with a smile? Your passion is what drives you forward.

•Variety Spice: Avoid being monotonous! Try some new online classes, apps, or exercise videos to liven things up. If you keep your mind and body active, boredom won't have an opportunity to flourish.

• Buddy Up: Invite a friend—real or imaginary—to go with you. Exercise becomes more enjoyable when there is mutual sweat and laughter, as well as accountability.

2.Establish Your Routine:

•Smart About Scheduling: Consider your exercises as significant appointments. Set out time on your calendar and honor it! Routine is the foundation of consistency, so choose a rhythm that suits you.

• Tiny Steps to Huge Success: Increase time and intensity little at first and then steadily. Honor accomplishments, no matter how little. Are you feeling overpowered? Recall that even ten minutes is preferable to none at all!

•Be Ready Like a Pro: The night before, arrange your training attire, tools, and water bottle. This easy step removes justifications and creates a smooth transition for commencing.

3.Transform it into a Lifestyle:

• Join the Dots: Incorporate activity throughout your day. You may dance during commercial breaks, perform squats while brushing your teeth, or use the stairs. Every little bit matters!

• Give yourself a reward: Honor your dedication! Enjoy a smoothie after your workout, a soothing bath, or a brand-new music selection for your training. Rewarding feedback maintains your motivation.

• Pay Attention to Your Body: Take breaks when needed! Injuries should never be forced to be endured. Prioritize your health, take pauses, and modify your workouts.

Recall that consistency is a process rather than a final goal. Although there will always be hiccups, the important thing is to keep moving forward and not to focus on perfection. Accept the enjoyment, acknowledge your little victories, and watch your at-home exercises turn into a happy, powerful experience!

Bonus Advice: Make your exercises into little journeys! Play entertaining fitness games, make your own routines, or discover new tracks. You'll stay longer the more you play!

Put on your sneakers, turn up the music, and go on a consistent and joyful adventure of home exercise!

COMMON STRUGGLES AND PLATEAUS

Ahh, the path to fitness! Exhilarating ascents, magnificent summits, and—gasp!—dreaded plateaus and bothersome struggles? Fear not, my fellow ascetic! Let's use some basic methods to get beyond those obstacles:

Challenge: Demotivation Crisis:

•Move: Determine your "why." Is it resilience, well-being, or just happiness? Bring the spark back to life by reminding yourself of your objectives and imagining your amazing future self.

• Add some zing! Are you in a rut? Modify your daily schedule! Take a fresh class, work out in the park, or dance to your own music selection. Inventiveness is your ally!

•Mini Wins Matter: Honor modest accomplishments! Have you completed a push-up yet? Take an additional minute to run? Give yourself a high five! Acknowledging even the smallest accomplishments refuels your motivation.

Plateau: The Condition of "Stuck in the Mud"

• Push Yourself: Increase the ferocity! Shorten rest intervals, raise rep counts, and add weights.

Your body yearns for fresh challenges in order to overcome that wall of plateauing.

•Switch It Up: Make your muscles confused! Experiment with various fitness routines, training approaches, and exercises. Sustain their curiosity to elicit fresh growth.

Fuel Smart: How much food do you eat? Eating a healthy diet is essential for both growth and healing. Make sure you're giving your body the nutrition it needs to meet your expectations.

Recall:

• Normal are plateaus: Remain calm! They serve as just brief stops for rest. Stay focused and have faith in the process.

• Pay attention to your body: It's never a good idea to push past pain. Take days off, and modify your exercise regimen as necessary.

• Honor the voyage: Take pleasure in the procedure! Put your attention on having fun, feeling well, and growing stronger. The outcomes will come next.

Bonus Tip: Monitor your advancement! To track your progress, utilize a fitness app or keep an exercise log. Seeing how much you've improved is a great incentive to keep going!

So, my fellow explorers, arm yourself with these easy-to-use tools, take on obstacles and plateaus head-on, and never give up on your fitness quest! It's an incredible view from the summit.

BEYOND WEIGHT LOSS

Let's chat about things other than weight reduction and put away the scale and rigid diets! It's time to adopt a comprehensive fitness philosophy that honors all the incredible things your body is capable of. This is the reason why:

Getting Past the Number:

•Strength & Power: Dispel the fallacy that "skinny = fit"! Concentrate on increasing your power, stamina, and strength. Feel the difference in your ability to climb, lift, and conquer!

•Mental Boost: Physical activity benefits your body as well as your mind! Reduce tension, improve attention, and experience an endorphin high. Feel more content, perceptive, and equipped to take on any task.

• Explosion of Confidence: Honor your body's amazing capabilities rather than focusing just on a scale. Feel powerful, capable, and self-assured in your own flesh.

• Long-Term Love: Sustainable living is more important than a short fix. Pay attention to lifelong healthy behaviors rather than ones you just adopt after you hit a particular weight.

Here are the items in your "Beyond Weight Loss" Toolkit:

•Reveal Your Joy: Do physical activities you enjoy! Explore new things, hike, swim, dance, and practice yoga. Make exercise an enjoyable activity rather than a chore.

•Fuel with Goodness: Give your body what it needs to feel alive and energized by nourishing it with tasty, healthful meals. Give up the diet mentality and adopt an awareness of your food.

• Honor Non-Scale Wins: Did you manage to run a little bit farther? Raise a greater weight? Enjoy your victories! Beyond only the scale's number, keep track of your advancement in other ways.

• Pay Attention to Your Body: Take breaks when necessary, and push yourself when you're ready. Give your body the respect it deserves and learn to trust its guidance.

•Discover Your Tribe: Assemble a supportive network of upbeat individuals around you. Make working out a happy experience for you both, set and discuss objectives, and celebrate each other's victories.

Recall:

Everybody has a unique journey. Avoid comparing yourself to other people and concentrate on your own special journey.

Take pleasure in the procedure. Exercise ought to be enjoyable, powerful, and enriching.

Honor each and every victory. Every accomplishment matters, whether it's more energy or deeper sleep.

Now let's go past the scale and into a realm where being fit means having a strong, self-assured, and capable sense of self. Accept the path, honor your physique, and achieve your objectives! When you pay attention to more than just a figure, the possibilities are infinite.

Adopt it as a way of life as a bonus! Include exercise and wholesome routines in your daily life. Make fitness a natural part of who you are; create nutritious foods, take the stairs.

BUILDING STRENGTH AND ENDURANCE

Put aside delicate blossoms, and let's develop into sturdy oak trees! Gaining strength and endurance is about more than simply looking beautiful, though that's a nice bonus! It's about giving oneself the ability to literally and figuratively climb any mountain. Here's how to accomplish it, simple as that:

Strength Bases:

•Bodyweight Buddies: Use your own body as the best gym by performing push-ups, squats, and lunges! If you can master these fundamentals, you'll lay a strong basis for learning more complex techniques.

• Iron Pals: You can be pals with weights! As you gain strength, progressively increase from a light start. Choose your playground: dumbbells, kettlebells, resistance bands!

•Progressive Play: Avoid being mired in a rut. Increase the number of repetitions, sets, or rest intervals to continue pushing your muscles and gaining gains.

Enhancers of Endurance:

•Cardio Champs: Pick an activity you like doing to get your heart rate up, such as bicycling, swimming, or running! Increase your distance and duration gradually.

•Vary Up Your Interval Adventures! Switch between short spurts of intense work and rest intervals. It burns a ton of calories and is similar to riding a roller coaster for your fitness.

•Go outside to work out in nature: this is your playground! Take a trail hike, a fast stroll, or a park game of tag. Your attitude and stamina are improved by landscape and fresh air.

Recall:

• Pay attention to your body: It's never a good idea to push through pain; rest when necessary.

•Fuel for Fire: Consume wholesome meals to provide your body with the energy it requires for growth and healing. Consider carbohydrates, protein, and good fats.

• Savor the process and celebrate the trip! Sensate the strength and endurance growing. Every stride is a triumph!

•Extra Advice: Locate an exercise partner! Training with a partner increases enjoyment, keeps you motivated, and allows you to appreciate each other's victories.

So let out your inner savage! With easy-to-implement yet powerful techniques, you may increase your strength, endurance, and fitness objectives. You are a formidable force, and the world is your gym!

HOME FITNESS FOR OVERALL WELL-BEING

Consider your house a launching pad rather than a gym! Exercise doesn't have to be limited to push-ups and squats; it may involve discovering a journey towards complete well-being. This is the reason why:

Physical Joy:

•**Strength & Confidence**: Develop the muscles necessary for daily strength and an internal confidence boost. Imagine climbing that flight of stairs or carrying groceries with ease!

•**Energy Explosion**: Forget about your midday slump! Your energy levels are boosted by exercise, making you feel energized and prepared to take on any task. Goodbye to lethargy and welcome to brightness!

•**Slayer of Stress**: Are you feeling overpowered? You may naturally reduce your stress by exercising. Moving about can help you achieve inner peace, relieve stress, and improve your attitude. Salutations to serenity!

Mental Magic:

• **Sharper Focus**: Prepare yourself for incredibly focused attention! Engaging in physical activity enhances cognitive abilities and memory, enabling you to be a productive employee or a star student in the classroom. Activate your brain power!

•**Sleep Symphony**: Having trouble falling asleep? Frequent exercise encourages sound sleep, making your bed into a comfortable haven where anxieties disappear. Sweet dreams are assured!

•**Emotional High**: Engaging in physical activity generates endorphins, which inherently elevate your mood and leave you beaming from ear to ear. Unleash the power of smiles!

Elevate Your Spirit:

• **Stress Management**: Do the obstacles of life feel too much to bear? Exercise gives you the tools to bounce back when things become rough by assisting with good stress management. Unlocking resilience!

•**Sense of Accomplishment**: No matter how minor the win, every workout counts. No matter how small your accomplishments may seem, acknowledge them and cultivate a strong feeling of self-worth. Confidence heightened!

•**Finding Joy:** Engage in things you genuinely love! Try yoga with your pet, swimming in the dawn, or dancing like nobody's watching. Turn exercising into a game rather than a job, and you'll feel so much better!
Recall:

•**Start Little, Dream Big**: Don't aim to transform into a superhero right away. Start with moderate exercise and progressively raise the length and intensity. The secret is to be consistent!

• **Pay Attention to Your Body**: Take breaks when necessary, and push yourself when you're ready. Honor the cues that your body gives you; it's a knowledgeable partner.

•**Make it Fun**: Let go of your drill sergeant attitude! Put on your favorite music, choose activities you enjoy, and host a fitness dance party at home. Having fun inspires motivation!

Bonus Advice: Be imaginative! While you wait for your coffee to brew, perform burpees, climb stairs for cardio, or perform lunges using furniture. Own your house, it's your gym!

So, let loose your inner fighter for wellbeing! Accept at-home exercise as a starting point for a more contented, healthy, and energetic you. The world is your playground, and the journey towards your well-being begins right now!

TRACKING PROGRESS

Keeping track of your progress is crucial to maintaining motivation and making sure you're on pace to meet your fitness objectives. It's important to pay attention to the changes in your body, mind, and general well-being rather than just the number on the scale. Here's how to keep a straightforward and efficient record of your progress:

1. Establish SMART objectives:

Make sure your goals are SMART—specific, measurable, achievable, relevant, and time-bound—before you begin tracking. This will support you throughout your fitness journey in maintaining motivation and focus.

2. Monitor Your Exercise:

To monitor your improvement, keep a workout log. This might involve your heart rate, the weights you lift, the length of your workouts, and the activities you perform.

3. Keep an eye on your body dimensions:

Make consistent measurements of your physique. Your body fat percentage, hip circumference, and waist circumference may be examples of this.

4. Evaluate Your Level of Energy:

Keep a journal of your feelings all day. Take note of your mood, energy level, and sleep quality.

5. Honor Non-Scale Triumphs:

Don't limit yourself to losing weight. Honor additional accomplishments like increasing your endurance, lifting bigger weights, or running a greater distance.

6. Employ trackers or apps for fitness:

You can monitor your progress with a variety of fitness trackers and apps. Tracking your exercises, body measurements, and other data may be made simple with these apps.

7. Let Others Know About Your Progress:

Maintaining accountability and motivation can be facilitated by discussing your achievements with loved ones, friends, or a workout partner.

8. Modify Your Strategy as Necessary:

Modify your exercise or diet regimen if you're not getting the desired results.

9. Don't Let Plateaus Discourage You:

Everybody occasionally reaches a plateau. If you follow your strategy, you will succeed in the end.

10. Savor the Trip:

Recall that achieving fitness is a process rather than a goal. Prioritize having fun during the process and implementing long-lasting, healthy lifestyle improvements.

Extra Advice:

Take pictures of your progress since it may be really inspiring to see the improvements in person.

Consider making progress videos. You can monitor your development and pinpoint areas for growth by keeping an eye on your own movements.

See a medical practitioner on a regular basis: They are able to monitor your general well-being and assist you in staying on course.

Recall that monitoring progress does not need perfection. It's about enjoying your progress along the road and adjusting as necessary. You can live a better, happier life and reach your fitness goals with commitment and perseverance!

MONITORING YOUR SUCCESS

In the world of at-home exercise, where staying motivated may be difficult and maintaining consistency is a never-ending struggle, tracking your progress is an essential tool for long-term success. You may maintain your motivation, concentration, and progress toward your fitness objectives by keeping track of your accomplishments, pinpointing your areas for growth, and acknowledging your accomplishments.

1. Determining Initial Measurements

Setting a benchmark for your current fitness level is crucial before starting any fitness program. This includes taking vital indicators including weight, body fat percentage, strength, flexibility, and endurance. As you advance, these baseline measures will be a useful point of comparison that will let you gauge how much you've improved and how successful your training has been.

2. Continually Assessing Development

After you've determined your baseline, it's important to begin routinely tracking your advancement. Depending on your interests and goals, this may entail check-ins every week, every two weeks, or every month. Regular monitoring gives you a clear view of your overall performance and assists you in identifying areas that could need more attention or modifications. Frequency is crucial.

3. Body Weight and Composition:

Although weight by itself doesn't provide a clear picture of one's level of fitness, it may be a helpful marker of changes in body composition. Regular self-weighing, preferably in the same settings, will enable you to monitor changes in your total weight. Additionally, think about utilizing calipers or a body fat scale to determine your body fat percentage. This gives you a more thorough evaluation of your body composition, taking into account the distribution of fat, lean body mass, and muscle mass.

4. Power and Sturdiness:

Incorporate progressive loading into your workouts to monitor your strength development. This entails escalating the weight or resistance you lift, the amount of repetitions, or the number of sets you complete gradually. You may evaluate your strength increases by keeping an eye on your capacity to perform more repetitions or manage bigger loads.

Time-based exercises or interval training may be used to track your development in endurance. When you see an improvement in your stamina over time, try to progressively increase the length or intensity of these exercises.

5. Adaptability

Although it's often disregarded in at-home workout regimens, flexibility is essential for preserving range of motion, lowering the risk of injury, and improving general health. Assess your flexibility on a regular basis by using instruments for flexibility evaluation or by executing routine stretches. Keep track of your progress by noting your reach or the ease with which you can do specific stretches.

6. Beyond Metrics: Honoring Significant Occurrences

Measuring success with metrics is vital, but it's just as crucial to acknowledge and reward non-numerical accomplishments. Take note of how your clothing fits better, how much more energy you have, or how much more confident you feel in day-to-day activities. These non-monetary benchmarks are just as significant and can serve as a source of inspiration.

7.Keeping an eye out for adaptation and consistency

It takes more than just data to measure your progress; you also need to know how your body reacts to your exercise routine. Regressions or plateaus are warning signs that you might need to modify your diet or workout regimen. To maintain your routine effective and challengingly, review your baseline data, evaluate your recent progress, and make any modifications.

In summary

A long-term home fitness quest requires regular success monitoring. It lets you recognize areas for growth, offers insightful information on how you're doing, and lets you celebrate your successes. You may confidently and enthusiastically overcome the obstacles of at-home fitness and accomplish your long-term objectives by regularly monitoring your metrics, identifying non-numerical milestones, and modifying your tactics in response to your input.

CELEBRATING MILESTONES

While reaching fitness objectives might be difficult, the road can also be very fulfilling. Celebrate your victories—big and small—along the journey to keep yourself inspired, give you more self-assurance, and highlight the benefits of your hard work. These little victories motivate you to keep going forward by giving you concrete proof of your progress and acting as stepping stones towards your ultimate goals.

1. Acknowledging Minor Triumphs

While achieving big goals like finishing a demanding exercise regimen or dropping a substantial amount of weight is undoubtedly something to celebrate, minor successes can have the biggest influence on your entire fitness journey. Celebrate the day you started exercising regularly, the day you learned a new workout method, or the week you were able to stick to a better diet. These little accomplishments, though they may not seem like much, represent important turning points in your life and should be recognized.

2. Acknowledging Non-Numerical Benchmarks

Fitness advancement goes beyond weighing readings and workout journals. Appreciate the changes in your life that you can celebrate, like having more energy, getting better sleep, or feeling better about the way you look. These non-gym-related achievements are frequently the most significant and visible, showing that improving general well-being rather than just numbers is the true goal of your fitness journey.

3. Establishing an Award Scheme

To recognize and celebrate your accomplishments, include a reward system in your workout regimen. This may be scheduling a fun activity, buying new exercise equipment, getting a massage, or just taking the day off to unwind and rejuvenate. These incentives encourage you to keep going after your fitness objectives by reinforcing the positive relationship with goal achievement.

4. Honoring the Community

Whether it's a supportive friend or family member, an online forum, or a group exercise class, share your fitness accomplishments with your fitness community. Not only does sharing your successes increase your personal sense of accomplishment, but it also motivates others and fosters a sense of community.

5. Festivities as Educational Chances

Any accomplishment, no matter how great or small, offers a chance to evaluate your development and pinpoint the factors that helped you succeed. Examine the workout regimens, dietary practices, and mental shifts that contributed to these successes. Make use of this knowledge to hone your strategy and establish new, even loftier objectives.

In summary

Celebrating accomplishments has a purpose beyond mere self-gratification: it serves to highlight the substantial impact of your hard work and to reaffirm your resolve to reach your fitness objectives. By celebrating your accomplishments, both large and little, monetary and non-monetary, you keep yourself motivated, build your self-esteem, and start a positive feedback loop that moves you closer to living a better and healthier lifestyle.

RESOURCES

Having the correct tools on hand may make all the difference in winning or losing the battle of home fitness, where there are many distractions and equipment constraints. This area provides you with a plethora of resources and information to enhance your training and achieve your objectives.

1. Constructing a Home Workout:

•Minimalist Must-Haves: Do not be discouraged by a lack of room. Yoga mats, bodyweight exercises, jump ropes, and resistance bands all provide effective workouts at a low cost.

• Cost-effective Upgrades: Stability balls, kettlebells, and dumbbells increase adaptability and provide increasing loading. Invest in long-lasting, high-quality items.

• Making the Most of Your Space: Wall-mounted racks, folding exercise equipment, and inventive storage options keep your exercise environment neat and clutter-free.

2. Nutritional Combat:

• Fueling Your Workouts: Recognize the significance of eating right before and after your workout. Find meal plans and dishes designed specifically for fans of at-home exercise.

• Hydration is Key: For the best possible performance and recuperation, it's important to stay hydrated both during the day and during physical activity. Examine some strategies for always having your water bottle close at hand.

• Overcoming Cravings: Acquire techniques to resist sugar cravings and make nutritious decisions without experiencing deprivation. Learn about meal suggestions and healthy snack alternatives.

3. Retaining Information and Motivation:

• Online communities and fitness apps: harness the power of technology! Look for applications that allow you to track your progress, receive individualized training plans, and interact with an online fitness community.

•Inspiring Books and Podcasts: Gain insight from other people's experiences. For inspiration, direction, and a good dose of motivation, engross yourself in fitness books and podcasts.

•Finding Your Tribe: To meet others who share your interests, sign up for online networks or neighborhood fitness organizations. Talking to others about your path can increase accountability and offer priceless support.

4. Beyond Fundamentals:

• Injury Prevention and Recovery: To avoid injuries, learn how to properly warm up, cool down, and pay attention to your body. Learn how to foam roll, stretch, and use other recovery strategies.

• Mental Toughness Training: Overcoming obstacles during exercise requires developing mental toughness. To maintain focus and win every set, use self-talk tactics, visualization exercises, and mindfulness practices.

• Time Management Tips: Balancing job, family, and health can be difficult. Learn time management strategies to squeeze in your exercises without compromising other commitments.

Recall that the ideal resources are those that meet your unique requirements and tastes. Try several things and see what suits you the best.

Your resource set will change as you go along, to meet your evolving fitness level and goals.

With the correct resources and information, you can fuel your path toward home fitness and witness your own success in overcoming obstacles. Warrior, the battleground is upon you!

RECOMMENDED EQUIPMENT

A world of accessibility and flexibility is made possible by home exercise, but it can be intimidating to navigate the equipment selection. "Strain Strategists" need not worry! This tutorial reveals everything you need to establish a strong home gym that fits your needs and budget.

The Essentials:

• Your Bodyweight: Your bodyweight is the best free tool available, providing countless exercise options. Strength and endurance may be developed without expensive equipment by modifying exercises like push-ups, squats, lunges, planks, and burpees to suit different skill levels.

•Resistance Bands: These adaptable devices, which come in a range of strengths, provide increasing resistance to an endless number of workouts that target every muscle area. They are lightweight, reasonably priced, and perfect for traveling or adding to bodyweight exercises.

•Yoga Mat: A yoga mat maximizes comfort and prevents injuries by offering padding and traction during floor exercises, stretches, and core training. To be even more environmentally conscientious, choose eco-friendly products.

•Jump Rope: A powerful aerobic exercise that increases heart rate, enhances coordination, and tones leg muscles. For an added effort, go for a weighted rope; alternatively, for short bursts of cardio, stay with a classic.

•Foam Roller: Your greatest buddy after a workout, a foam roller helps with recuperation, flexibility, and the release of tense muscles. Roll out painful areas for a few minutes, allowing the knots to release.

Bonus Equipment for Focused Training:

• Kettlebells and dumbbells: Free weights increase training intensity and muscle mass. When you gain strength, gradually raise the weight from the lighter starting point. Kettlebells test core stability, whereas dumbbells are more versatile.

• Pull-Up Bar: This equipment installed in doorways releases upper body strength. Beginners can master assisted variants, while experts can do sophisticated pull-ups and chin-ups.

•Suspension Trainer: Attach this adaptable device to a door or strong beam to work various muscle groups simultaneously in dynamic exercises. Ideal for houses with limited space or for vacation.

•Stability Ball: By adding instability to workouts, this inflated sphere strengthens your core and enhances your balance. Use it to give your training a fun twist by using it for planks, bridges, and core rotations.

•Medicine Ball: Adding diversity and explosive force to your routine, you may roll, smash, or throw the medicine ball. With this adaptable tool, you may increase core strength, improve coordination, and raise your heart rate.

Recall that equipment is only a tool. Your dedication, consistency, and "Strain Strategist" mentality are the keys to success. No matter the size of the gym, if you concentrate on good form, gradual overload, and a well-rounded program, you'll achieve your goals.

Pro Tip: Put more money on quality than quantity. Select sturdy, adaptable gear that can meet your changing exercise requirements. To get the most out of your workout and prevent injuries, research safety precautions and appropriate form.

One strain at a time, start with your essentials, add more as your demands change, and take on your at-home fitness adventure!

CONCLUSION

You've overcome the obstacles, perspired through the exercises, and rejoiced in your victories. Now that your at-home fitness adventure has reached its peak, it's time to take stock of your progress and reinforce your accomplishments. Not only has the Strain Strategist Approach helped you lose weight, but it has also opened a new chapter in your overall health and wellbeing. Together, let's review the tenets that brought you here and explore the countless opportunities that await.

Summary of the Approach of the Strain Strategist:

•Pay attention to the "big three"—cardiovascular endurance, strength, and flexibility—as they are the foundations of a strong and flexible body.

•Accept Gradual Overload: Gradually push your boundaries to make sure you're always challenged and developing.

•Pay attention to your body's needs. To prevent injury, emphasize good form, accept rest days, and adjust to obstacles.

•Fuel from nutrition: Fill your body with healthy nutrients to maximize function and recuperation.

•Moving with mindfulness: Turn exercise into a self-awareness practice by developing a connection with your body and movements.

Your Route to Success in Home Fitness and Beyond:

With the knowledge and resources provided by The Strain Strategist, you can confidently navigate the home fitness scene. But the adventure doesn't stop after you accomplish your first objectives.

Here's how to maintain the momentum:

•Variety is essential. Try out various training methods, such as yoga or HIIT, to avoid plateaus and create enthusiasm.

•Create fresh obstacles: Achieve personal bests, longer endurance achievements, or master difficult exercises to push your limits.

•Community issues: Seek out like-minded people in person or online for motivation, support, and a common interest in fitness.

•Beyond reducing weight: Accept the all-encompassing advantages of exercise, such as better sleep, increased stress tolerance, and a fresh understanding of your body's potential.

•Transform it into a way of life: Whether it's walking through the outdoors, dancing to your favorite music, or using the stairs, include movement into your everyday routine.

You now have the ability to take charge of your health and lay the groundwork for a lifetime of wellbeing thanks to The Strain Strategist. Recall that there is a continuous, not a linear, road to success. Keep pursuing the thrill of activity, accept new challenges, and celebrate your accomplishments. Now that you've discovered home fitness's actual potential, the options are virtually limitless.

Proceed with self-assurance, driven by your acquired knowledge and expertise. The Strain Strategist has prepared you for the road, but it is up to you to create the next chapters of your fitness narrative—one exercise, one step, and one victorious breath at a time.

REVIEW PAGE

Dear Reader,

I hope this communication finds you well. I'm writing to express my heartfelt appreciation for exploring "The Strain Strategist: Home Fitness for Weight Loss and Beyond." Your dedication to your fitness quest is very admirable.

As an author, feedback from readers like you is vital in creating and improving future editions. I would be thankful if you could take a few seconds to express your opinions on the book. Your candid feedback will not only help me understand what resonated with you, but it will also benefit others contemplating this book for their fitness aspirations.

Whether you found the information informative, have recommendations for improvement, or simply want to share your personal experience, your feedback is much appreciated. You may submit your review.

Thank you for becoming a member of the "The Strain Strategist" community once more. Your comment helps the continuous journey of assisting folks in achieving their fitness goals through efficient home exercises.

I wish you the best of luck on your fitness quest!

Warm regards,

Meta J.Myers